I0785452

BOOST YOUR IMMUNE SYSTEM

Michal Kloczkowski

Copyright © 2012 Michal Kloczkowski
All rights reserved.
ISBN:1979068798
ISBN-13:978-1979068798

CONTENTS

ACKNOWLEDGMENTS

Special thanks to friend of mine Ed Fountaine. We spent hours talking about health benefits of plant-based diet. He shared some valuable insights with me. This encouraged me to write this book, so other people can take great care of their health.

CHAPTER ONE

MY STORY

I was in my early twenties and my **immune system was very weak**. I was getting a cold, flue, runny nose or sore throat at least once a month. Every day I wake up tired after eight hours of sleep feeling no energy throughout the day. One winter I suffer from the flue for four weeks. This experience tells me only one thing. I have to do something about it. I go to the doctors and get the flue jab. It doesn't really help. I still get ill. The only difference is the symptoms are not as severe as before. This is not what I want. I'm thinking of what else I can do to **boost my immune system** and stop getting ill so often. I doubt that this is possible. I blame my genes for this. One day I am having a conversation in my house with my best friend about it. My friend tells me about the book The pH Miracle written by Dr. Robert Young. He says to me "this book is about the diet and if you follow it you will never get ill again". I'm reading this book and there are stories of people who recovered from mental diseases and cancer. I find it hard to believe what I am reading. The only way to find out if it is true or not, is to try it.

This is how my journey to achieve perfect health began.
I invested time in reading books and watching seminars
to gain the knowledge and understanding about how our
bodies function at the physical level, and what we eat,
drink, think and believe in affects our health and our
well-being. The hardest part was to put all of this
knowledge in to practice and stay motivated.

I am passionate about helping people to live a healthy
life. I decided to write this book because it makes me
feel sad when I see people eating unhealthy food and
then getting ill. They suffer from diseases caused by bad
food choices and later they wonder why they got this
disease or that disease. Yet nobody makes the
connection between food choices and diseases. They run
to the doctor hoping that he or she will somehow help
them but in reality, if it is terminal illness or chronic
disease the result is miserable suffering or even death.
In both cases, ill people suffer as well as their families.
The worst thing is when children die from cancer or
suffer from diabetes. When I hear about cases like this I
scream inside me and wonder how this is possible that a
four-year-old gets diabetes or cancer and then dies. They
are illnesses of old people. Children shouldn't get them. I
want to teach you to take responsibility for your health
and well-being and to make better food and lifestyle
choices that prevent this from happening to you and
your family. It is time to take responsibility for your
health so your loved ones don't have to watch you

suffering and dying. It's time to take responsibility for you and your family's health so you don't have to see members of your family, including your children suffering and dying from illness. It's easy to prevent all of this. Actually, it's easier than you think it is. It's a **Plant-Based Food Diet** that can prevent most of the nasty diseases and even reverse some of them. The most difficult part is to change your attitude and mindset and I will help you with this. I will guide you. I am not a doctor I will simply share my knowledge and experience with you.

Shortly after going 100% plant-based I felt so much better. I felt more energetic. My skin looked better. I noticed an improvement in the quality of my hair. I look younger than I am. I lost 10 kilograms in 2 weeks. The most important thing is that my immune system improved. I don't get ill, not even the flu, or colds etc. I remember the last time I was Ill was in December 2010 when I was still in my transition period. I tested it on myself and I knew it's working so I didn't see any point in going back to my old eating habits and feeling sluggish most of the time or getting ill every so often.
This change gave me peace of mind because I realized that I dropped chances significantly to get cancer, diabetes, heart attack or other nasty diseases.

I proved to myself that impossible is possible if you really want it, and if you believe that you can do it.

CHAPTER TWO

Benefits of Plant-Based Food Diet

1. Lower Risk of Getting Cancer

The research shows that a diet reach in meat and dairy may quadruple the risk of getting this nasty disease. Obviously, you also have to try to avoid smoking and alcohol. The best way to decrease the chance of getting cancer is to completely eliminate animal proteins and animal fat from your diet and go on a Plant-Based Diet.

In the book, The China Study author is saying about Indian researches who studied two groups of rats. The first group was given cancer-causing aflatoxin and fed a diet that was composed of 20% animal protein. Every single animal developed liver cancer. In the second group, animals were given this same amount of aflatoxin, but this time a fed diet that was only composed of 5% animal protein. The second group didn't develop liver cancer.

2.   Lower Risk of Getting Diabetes

<u>Consuming plant protein reduces the risk of getting type 2 diabetes.</u> Dr. Neal Bernard explains in his <u>book</u> <u>The Scientifically Proven System for Reversing Diabetes</u> that diabetes is caused by the combination of sugar in your blood and animal fat in your cells. In a healthy person sugar, with the help of insulin would enter the cell to give you energy, and eventually would be removed from the body, but animal fat prevents this transition. Sugar stays in your bloodstream. High levels of sugar in your bloodstream are toxic to your body. Your doctor tells you that you have high levels of glucose in your blood, and the next thing you know is that you are diagnosed with diabetes.

3.   Weight Loss

We've been told that to lose weight we have to lose fat. We load our bodies with toxins and make it acidic by the food we eat. Our bodies defence mechanism tries to keep toxins away from the vital organs by storing them in fat. If you want to lose weight you don't want to lose fat you want to lose toxins and acid from your body. You can do that by consuming a whole foods, plant-based diet, especially one that is low in fat and processed sugar. In fact try to avoid processed sugar as it is very toxic to our bodies and makes our bodies acidic. Remember that other kinds of processed food, meat and dairy products also make your body acidic. Eat food that makes your body alkaline and flush acid and toxins out of your body. Dr. Robert Young explains in depth this problem in his book "The pH Miracle for weight loss". After reading this book you will look differently at the food you eat.

4. Boost Your Immune System

As I mentioned earlier I used to get ill very often. One day I came across the book <u>The pH Miracle</u>. Basically, the book was saying that if the pH of your body is below 7 that means that your body is acidic. The lower the pH is, the more acidic your body is. An acidic body is unhealthy body full of toxins. Your immune system is not working properly. You are very likely to get ill. An acidic body is a perfect environment for bad bacteria and disease to develop. On the other hand if the pH of your body is above 7 that means that your body is alkaline. An alkaline body is a healthy body. Your immune system is boosted. You are unlikely to get ill. Even though you get infected by bacteria or a virus the disease won't develop in your body as long as it remains alkaline. To understand it better imagine a swimming pool. If they don't put chemicals in the water to keep the pH of the water above 7 meaning alkaline, soon mould would grow. The mould, bacteria is already in the water but the only thing which prevents it from growing is alkalinity of the water. This same rule applies to your body.

How to measure pH of your body?

The ideal pH of the body is slightly alkaline 7.30-7.45. You can test your pH levels by using litmus paper in your saliva or urine first thing in the morning before eating or drinking anything.

5.   Lower Blood Pressure

Eating a plant-based diet will help you with high blood pressure because you are consuming foods rich in potassium. Too much sodium causes high blood pressure. <u>The more potassium you eat, the more sodium you lose through urine</u>.

How to Keep Your Body Healthy

From the above chapter, you know that to achieve optimum health and prevent diseases you have to keep the pH of your body between 7.30 and 7.45. How do you do this? It's very easy. You have to stop eating foods which make your body acidic, are full of toxins and preservatives and start eating unprocessed whole foods that make your body alkaline. In chapter 4 you will find out which foods make our bodies acidic and therefore you are prone to get ill, feeling tired sluggish etc. In chapter 5 you will find out how to keep your body alkaline, and therefore healthy. A healthy body means you feel more energetic, you are unlikely to get ill even though people around you suffer from flue and cold. Disease won't develop because your body is alkaline and your immune system is boosted. You decrease a chance to get cancer, diabetes and other nasty disease. Doesn't it sound great? Read it on.

CHAPTER FOUR

Foods Which Make Your Body Acidic

I do not eat products listed below not because I can't, I don't want to. I know it is bad for my body, so I don't want to eat it. There is a big difference in perception between I can't and I don't want to.

- _Refined White Sugar_ – It makes your body acidic. In other words its decreases the pH of your body. You can find sugar in processed foods such as pasta, ketchup, yogurt, fizzy drinks etc. Over consuming sugar can contribute to diabetes, tooth decay, obesity and candida overgrowth. I recommend you use stevia instead, which is a natural sweetener, and an alternative to sugar. Other natural sweeteners which are highly processed are Agave Nectar, Molasses.

- _Artificial Sweeteners_ – They are worse than sugar. They are very acidifying. Aspartame is the worst, one of the ingredients, methyl alcohol, converts into formaldehyde, a deadly neurotoxin. Artificial sweeteners can cause symptoms such as headaches, migraines, depression, heart palpitation, seizures, fatigue, weight gain, anxiety, muscle spasm, epilepsy, mental retardation, Alzheimer's. Please check the packaging for ingredients before you purchase or consume any product.

- _Processed Foods_ – Try to avoid eating any processed food as they contain sugar and other preservatives which are harmful to our bodies. Let's say I want to cook something where the main ingredient is kidney beans, I do not buy them in the tin, I buy them in the bag, soak them overnight, and then cook them. Try to eat wholefoods. An apple is a wholefood.

- _Meats and Eggs_ – Yes they as well make your body acidic. They are filled with hormones, antibiotics, mycotoxins, steroids and the saturated fats that contribute to heart disease, stroke and cancer.

- _Milk and Dairy Products_ – Most mainstream health organisations recommend that you consume 2-3 servings per day. My friends, I am here to tell you why it is bad for you to consume them. Let's start with an obvious thing. Cows' milk is designed for baby cows, whose requirements are far different from those of humans. Secondly, dairy products contain hormones, antibiotics and saturated fat. The main protein in milk is called Casein and is **TOXIC** to humans. It is therefore responsible for eczema, acne, kidney disease, irritable bowel syndrome, sinus problems. There is more calcium in broccoli than in the cow's milk. You can use alternatives. Almond milk, rice milk etc.

Note: Citric fruits have low pH however they don't have a bad effect on your body like the products listed above. Fruits such as lemon, lime or grapefruit have no sugar in them, so it has an alkalising effect on your body.

CHAPTER FIVE

Ways of Making Your Body Alkaline

I do eat products listed below not because I have to, I want to. I know it is good for my body, and I want to eat it. Again there is a big difference in the perception. Focus more on what you want to eat, rather than on what you don't want to eat.

- _Vegetables and Fruits_ — Just try to eat lots of vegetables as they will quickly detoxify and make your body alkaline. Eat moderate amount of fruits because they contain sugar. If you eat too many carbohydrates you may put on weight. If you are trying to lose weight try to decrease the amount of carbohydrates you consume.

- _Juicing_ — The best way to nourish and make your body alkaline is to drink green juices or smoothies. On the website juicerecipes.com you will find juices for weight loss and for health. It's amazing what juices can do for your health. They will clean your whole body, blood, tissues, organs, intestinal tract (perfect if you suffer from constipation). Let's say you suffer from a particular health condition, click on the tab marked "health" and find recipes that could help. If you are allergic or you don't like any of the ingredients in the recipe just don't add it to your juice. It's not a big deal. If you don't have a slow juicer you can still drink green smoothies. Just try not to make smoothies only made out of fruits, add some vegetables as well such us spinach, carrot, beetroot etc.

- *Lemon or Lime Water* – Drink a glass of lemon or lime water. Even though it contains citric acid it has an alkalising effect on your body. Drinking lemon water on a daily basis for a certain period of time will help you to boost your energy and mood, lose weight, rejuvenate skin, aid digestion and detoxification.

- *Organic Apple Cider Vinegar* – see the chapter below.

CHAPTER SIX

Organic Apple Cider Vinegar

Organic Apple Cider Vinegar thanks to its compounds such as magnesium, potassium, acetic acid, enzymes and probiotics it has so many amazing health benefits that I decided to write a whole chapter on this.

Makes Our Body Alkaline

Acetic acid, even though it is an acid, has an alkalising effect on the rest of your body. It reduces the risk of getting chronic diseases like cancer or diabetes.

It works like a natural antibiotic without side effects

Acetic acid has the ability to kill "bad" bacteria and at this same time promotes the growth of "friendly" bacteria. As a result, it promotes healthy digestion, boosts your immune system, improves your skin and hair.

Helps To Lose Weight

Apple cider vinegar promotes weight loss because it kills your hunger and cravings. It also reduces your body fat and increases your metabolism.

Lowers Blood Pressure

It lowers your blood pressure thanks to its high potassium content.

Kills Candida (Yeast Infection)

Bacteria called candida is normally found in the gastrointestinal tract. We would die without it. However, if your body is acidic it can easily become drastically overgrown, causing a wide variety of symptoms from annoying to chronic to fatal such as fatigue, indigestion, food cravings, poor memory, colds and flues, muscle aches, ulcers. This is only to name a few. Read the book The pH Miracle to find out more about candida.

Can Detox Your Body

It removes harmful toxins from your blood, tissues, lungs and liver. It basically cleanses your whole body.

How to Take It

Consume up to 1 tablespoon with water, preferably before meals. If it's too much for you decrease the amount to for example 1 teaspoon. Because everybody is different, experiment on yourself to see how much you can take.

CHAPTER SEVEN

YOUR HEALTH

From the above chapter, you know that I used to be a very unhealthy person eating unhealthy food, thinking it is pretty much healthy but I was wrong. In fact, I knew nothing about being healthy and most importantly I didn't know how it feels to be perfectly healthy. I didn't know how it feels to be free from the worry of getting one of those nasty diseases. I invested time in educating myself, and I took the necessary steps to apply the knowledge into my life. I felt great about it. I lost weight, felt more energetic, and most importantly I stopped getting ill every so often. That's enough about me. I have already helped myself. Now I want to help you. Let's talk about you.

It's not just a healthy diet which you do for some time and then you go back to where you were. It's a healthy lifestyle which will benefit you in the long run. In order to become a super healthy person who lives a healthy lifestyle day in, day out and is an example for others to follow, you must **take responsibility for your health**.

Below you can see the mindset and habits of a person who takes responsibility for their health:

1. _Person who takes responsibility for their health_ **puts their health as number one priority.** If you have a family then health for all of you should be your number one priority.

2. _Person who takes responsibility for their health_ **constantly educates himself or herself about a healthy lifestyle and healthy eating**. For example by reading books (don't forget to apply the knowledge in your life). I recommend you to read The pH Miracle or China Study. This is necessary to get a deeper understanding of how your body works and what to do to achieve optimum health. You don't stop by reading just one book. You try to get information from other sources, for example, YouTube or maybe you will find someone who is already doing it to share your knowledge and experience with them. You can have a really good and interesting conversation.

Note:

I mentioned and explained a little bit about the benefits of a plant-based diet in the above chapters. I encourage you to read one of those books because they were written by doctors who were specialists in their field. I'm not a doctor. I'm here to share my experience with you and tell you that a healthy life without fear of getting nasty diseases is possible.

Back to the topic.

3. *Person who takes responsibility for their health* **treats their body like a temple** by making the best food choices.

4. *Person who takes responsibility for their health* **DOES NOT** treat their body like an amusement park by eating everything like a pig.

5. Needless to say that *Person who takes responsibility for their health* **DOES NOT** eat junk food and avoids fast-foods.

6. *Person who takes responsibility for their health* **DOES NOT** buy or eat processed foods.

7. *Person who takes responsibility for their health* eats **whole unprocessed foods.**

8. *Person who takes responsibility for their health*, if possible, **buys produce in their local store**.

9. *Person who takes responsibility for their health* learns how to say **NO** to people (even if they are family members or friends) when they are offered something they don't want to eat.

10. _Person who takes responsibility for their health_ **DOES NOT** think: I can't eat a chocolate bar, ice-cream (both are full of refined sugar) instead a health mentality person thinks: I don't want to eat it because I know that is unhealthy for me.

11. _Person who takes responsibility for their health_ **checks the ingredients of the product before the purchase.** If one of the ingredients is refined sugar or artificial sweetener such as aspartame do not touch it.

CHAPTER EIGHT

Putting It Together

You already educated yourself, you have done some research and you made a conscious decision to take responsibility for your health. You want to eat healthy but for some reason, you can't.

You may say: "this diet is very healthy but it's so difficult to do because of this and that" or "what worked for you might not work for everybody" or "I don't have time". What you are really saying is: "I'm not willing to give the time and effort necessary to make it work for me". You don't believe in yourself that you can make it against all the odds and obstacles. In fact, there is only one obstacle you have to overcome. Yes, it's you and your perception and belief system about yourself. Yes, you are absolutely right it is difficult. Good news is I'm here to help you to make it easier..

Just......

Believe that you can do it. Believe in yourself.

Find out **what is your "why"**. What is your heart desire? For example "I want to prevent and avoid illnesses and live a long healthy life".... Or ... "I want to lose weight" .....or.... "I want to be free from cold, flu and headaches"... etc.

Once you know what your heart's desire is, **create a vision for your life of being healthy**, instead of setting up another goal. Why? Because vision has the higher purpose. Vision is the "why". What you want to get out of your life and how you envision your life. That means you look at your core values and beliefs and you are willing to change them in order to achieve it. You identify yourself with your new healthy lifestyle. It's not going to be easy but it's going to be a fantastic journey which will change your life for the better.

Remember that vision without action is a dream.

Speaking of action. If you can go from eating "junk" food to vegan plant-based diet in one day. Congratulations! I couldn't do it. **I needed a 5 month transition period when I was teaching myself how to make healthy food** (see links with recipes in chapter recipes). Everybody is different, you may need less or more time then I needed. You may develop another strategy to achieve it. Whatever you do, be consistent, and never lose focus and faith in yourself.

Everyday think about what steps you can take to become healthier person. Think what would you have for breakfast that is healthy. Educate yourself first so you have an idea what is really healthy what is not.

Take baby steps to give up what is bad for your body. For example, first give up refined sugar than milk and meat.

Take baby steps to **develop healthy eating habits**. At the beginning try to add more vegetables to each meal you eat. Later you may realise that food you eat in a canteen in your workplace is not good. Bring food you make at home to eat it at work.

So many people want to make changes, for example, lose weight and they never actually start doing it or they quit half way through or they don't do the right thing to achieve it. Do not rely on your motivation because it's never around when you need it. Don't take me wrong I'm not saying that motivation is something bad. Don't rely only on motivation. **Try to build healthy habits and mindset**. Learn to check the ingredients of the product before you purchase it. Learn how to prepare healthy meals. Learn how to plan your healthy meals. Learn how to plan your shopping. If you want to eat healthy you have to plan your shopping and your meals few days ahead.

You must stay focused. Never forget that you want to live a healthy life. When you are thinking about it **believe that you can achieve it**.

CHAPTER NINE

Mental-Movie, Affirmations and Health

I would like to elaborate more on the subject of people wanting to make changes in their life or achieving their goals but for one reason or the other, they are not able to do it. As you may know, we have two kinds of minds: conscious mind and subconscious. You may want to do something consciously but if your subconscious mind doesn't want it, you're not going to achieve it. You may not even take the first step. You may procrastinate. To prevent this from happening the conscious and subconscious mind must be aligned.

How to do this?

In your mind create a mental – movie. See yourself being healthy, losing weight, recovering from illness, headaches etc. This way you send the signal to the subconscious mind that this what you want. This is the direction you want your life to go. I can't stress enough that this mental picture held in your mind must be backed up with faith and the subconscious mind will bring it to pass. You should feel joyful and restful while imagining this in your mind. Also feel the reality of it. Find a quiet place or room. Sit on your chair or lay dawn in the bed, relax your body and start to create pictures of your mental -movie. Do it if you can twice or three times a day. If you can do it only once a day that's fine too. **Believe in yourself. Believe that you can achieve it**. Go easy on yourself. Do not tie your happiness to your goal. Do not try too hard. If you try too hard you put pressure on your subconscious mind and it doesn't like it when you do that and you may get the opposite result to that which you want. During or after visualization feel that you already achieved that. If you don't know how it feels, ask yourself a question. "How it feels to be super healthy?" and notice if something has changed how you feel about it.

 Let me emphasize that mental images you make in your mind are very powerful. Let's say you want to give up smoking, you may manage to stop smoking for some time, but if you are still making images of you enjoying it, you're going to come back to where you were. If you focus on something you don't want, you get what you don't want because you use your imagination against yourself. Use your imagination in your favour by focusing on what you want.

Affirmations are another technique you can use to help you to go on a plant-based diet.

Affirmations are positive, specific statements that help you overcome self-sabotaging, negative thoughts. They help you make positive changes in your life. Some examples of affirmations:

- "I am so happy and grateful that now I eat healthy".
- "I am so happy and grateful that now I am on a plant-based diet".
- "I have lost weight on a plant-based diet".
- "I'm free from food cravings".

 Keep them short and positive. Affirmations should be formed in the present tense. Again find a quiet room and try to relax your body. Repeat affirmations at least five times in a row. While repeating those statements do not use vain repetition. Know what you are saying and why you are saying it. Listen to what you are saying. If necessary pause for few seconds so your mind can accept the idea. Believe in what you are saying.

CHAPTER TEN

Removing Mental Obstacles

<u>The two above techniques would work very well If you overcome the following obstacles:</u>

1. Negative Believes

You may believe that you cannot survive without eggs, meat, milk and dairy. You may believe that those foods are healthy because they contain proteins, calcium and vitamins. Which is a true, they do contain vital minerals and vitamins, we need (You can find all of vitals minerals and vitamins in plants). If you use common sense you would think those foods are healthy. The trick is, you don't see the whole picture. Do you remember the story with experiment on rats? Do you remember what I told you about milk and dairy in above chapter?

The best way to change this beliefs is to educate yourself by reading books(I recommend <u>The pH Miracle</u> , <u>The China Study</u>, <u>Eat To Live</u> or <u>The Scientifically Proven System for Reversing Diabetes</u>) and blogs(<u>Dr. Michael Greger</u> or <u>Dr. Barnards Blog</u>) or watching Youtube Videos.

 I'm not saying that you have to belife in every word I said only because I said so or someone else said so. Once you get the knowledge, test it on yourself, as I did and see if you feel better. You need to alllow some time (more and less three moths) before you can say if its working for you or not.

2. Negative Thoughts And Voices In Your Head

If you have negative thoughts or a little voice in your head is telling you something like "you can't do it …or … it's not worth it"…. Or… "it's too difficult to do it" … or….. "you will die anyway so there is no point to eat healthy"… etc. Do not give them any power by dwelling on them, arguing with them, reasoning with them, or fighting them. You cannot stop this little voice in your head talking to you but you can choose not to listen to it. Imagine a volume nob and turn it down and do what you have to do.

3. Doubt

Don't let doubts get into your head. If the doubt creeps up, be aware of it, relax and let it go. Easier said than

done? Let me give you some practical advice. Identify it and say goodbye to it as you would to your old and good friend. To your surprise, it may dissolve and go away. If it doesn't that means you are not ready to let it go because you want it. It's part of your identity and you can't imagine living without it. You are not ready to change yet.

4. Food Craivings

Food craving is an intense desire to consume a specific food. One part of you knows it is unhealthy, the other part of you really want it, you can't help it, you eat it you feel bad afterwards.

To win this battle friend of mine uses following strategy(please try not to laugh or he will be upset):

Whenever he craves food, he takes a bite and chews food for as long as he can before he feels like he has no choice but to swallow it and then spits it out. That way he tricks his brain, he satisfies his food cravings without eating it and causing damage to his body.

Are you sweet tooth? If you are craving for sweet-tasting food, try to take a spoon of sugar into your mouth. I wonder how long can you hold it for before you spit it out.

Do you have meat craving? Try to chew raw meat or imagine is raw(if it's not). I bet you won't be putting it

into your mouth any more. You will be like: ewww…….. meat is so disgusting.

4. Fear of Being Criticazed

I often hear people saying something like "I would like to go vegan (plant based-diet is basically a vegan diet) but I can't because of the people around me".

 One friend told me "I've watched the movie <u>WHAT THE HEALTH</u> (Also available on Netflix). It was a real eye-opener for me but when I told people that I am thinking about going vegan they looked at me and they said I am crazy".

I told him not to look for people's approval because this need for approval will hold him back, create anxiety, stop him from doing important things, and he will never achieve his dream of being healthy.

I also told him not to let someone else's opinion make him feel bad about himself. I said "learn how to accept criticism, whatever you do there will be always someone who will criticise you".

People who criticize you for going vegan have no clue about eating healthy. They may think they are experts on nutrition, but they have no idea.

I also mentioned to my friend "don't let anybody steal your dreams away from you". If someone says something like "you shouldn't do that because of this and that" or … "are you crazy? this is stupid idea" … and you end up not doing it. They have stolen a dream away from you. The worst thing is that you let them do it.

If you eliminate above obstacles it would make the transition much easier for you.

CHAPTER ELEVEN

Final Thoughts

I know what you may think right now. This diet takes too much time and effort. If you can't find time to eat healthy now, you will have to find time for illnesses later. Before becoming vegan, I thought that cooking takes to much time. From time to time I wanted to cook something, but I never had a time. So I end up not doing it. I realised I was wasting lots of time in front of TV or laptop. I was not doing anything productive. I decided to stop watching TV and spend less time in front of a laptop. Miraculously I found time to prepare healthy meals.

Before I became vegan I didn't even like cooking. All changed when I started my "vegan" journey. I can exactly explain what happened. Maybe at the bottom of my heart, I felt that vegan plant-based diet it's a right food for my body, mind and spirit and I simply followed my heart's desire.

If you "fall off the wagon" don't feel guilty or down, forgive yourself and simply get back on again.

This diet requires self-discipline. "Self-discipline is an ability to give yourself command and follow it". Command yourself that you gonna be healthy and do everything to make it happen. Be patient and consistent.

The most common question people ask me is "where do you get your protein from?"

Well… There is plenty of protein in plants and even in some fruits. You can't be protein deficient. So don't worry about not getting enough protein. Think of getting enough nutrients from the food you eat.

You see most people are deficient in zinc and magnesium. A lack of those two minerals is very common. Zinc will boost your immune system and it will help to protect you against infections such as the common cold. Zinc is also an important mineral that acts as a co-factor for over 200 metabolic enzymes. Magnesium is also important for the function of over 300 enzymes, and its vital for every major metabolic reaction from the synthesis of protein and genetic material to the production of energy from glucose. From my one experience, I recommend that you take zinc or magnesium in liquid form as they absorb very quickly.

Do not expect that you will become a healthy person in one hour, or after eating just one or two healthy meals. Life is not a Hollywood movie. You won't become healthy overnight. Especially after years of "abusing" your body, the temple and home for your soul. It will take sometime and persistence.

I wish you a fantastic journey. I hope you will make your health your number 1 priority. I hope that taking responsibility for your health will be a life changing experience for you and your family (If you have one).

Lastly, you should not feel sad, bad, overwhelmed, powerless or ashamed because you want to live a healthy life. You should feel happy, excited, and proud because you want to live a healthy life.

Remember you eat to live and thrive, you don't live to eat (shit food) and then die (from illnesses).

 Follow me on <u>Facebook</u> (HWBCOUCH) if you want me to help you to live a healthy life. I will show you what to eat and not to eat to be super healthy. Its so easy to be healthy.

I'm more than happy to receive any feedback or comments. Do not hesitate to contact me on <u>healthmentality@gmail.com</u>, and tell me how I can improve it to provide more value to readers.

Recipes

http://www.onegreenplanet.com has a massive collection of recipes and is a great source for veganising favourite recipes
Simple recipes:

http://www.minimalistbaker.com

recipes for those on a budget:

http://plantbasedonabudget.com/

http://www.ilovevegan.com/resources/vegan-lifestyle-on-a-budget/

https://www.youtube.com/channel/UCEjkioV3LO_OIUaSWRxFZ3A/featured

http://www.veggieonapenny.com/

gluten free and sugar free on a budget:

http://www.nothymetolose.com/

More gluten-free and other allergies:

http://ohsheglows.com/ (has an allergy section)

https://simplygluten-free.com/gluten-free-recipes/vegan

Indian and creative recipes:

http://www.veganricha.com

very popular:

http://www.buddhistchef.com

ABOUT THE AUTHOR

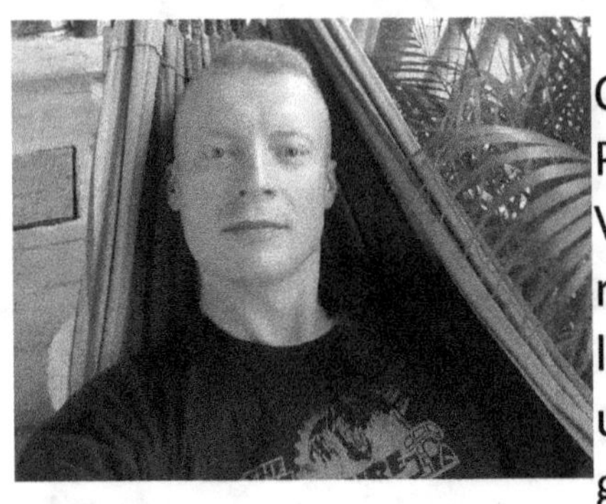

My name is Michal. Originally I come form Poland. I live in the UK now. Veganism changed my life so much and probably saved my life too. I used to be very unhealthy person, prone to get ill every month. After changing to vegan **plant-based diet** I reclaimed my health. It was a beautiful journey because apart from changing my eating habits I also had to change my mindset. I had to open my mind and heart to new knowledge about healthy eating and put the knowledge into practice. My whole life changed. Now heath is my number one priority.

Thanks to veganism I became more compassionate and empathetic towards animals. I mean all animals pets and farm animals who are being abused and killed in millions on daily basis.

Every year I set up for adventure usually in faraway countries. When I am there I like to spend some time in nature.

In my free time, I like to go to the gym, yoga classes. In the summer I like to go for bike rides with friends.

Thank you for reading my book.

Treat your body like temple.

www.ingramcontent.com/pod-product-compliance
Lightning Source LLC
Chambersburg PA
CBHW070100260726
48658CB00002B/924